Dedication: I dedicate this book to sincere lovers of art who seek to cultivate their greatest asset, which is the health of body and mind, and who think about honoring traditions.

Santarém, December 19, 2024
Sifu Zeca da Vila Barbosa (Lai Hop Long)

Introduction

In ancient times, during difficult times, it was common for families to send their children to the Shaolin temple to study and eat.
A child was taken by his father to Shaolin. The child, who was about 6 years old, dedicated himself to studying and the hard Shaolin training for six months. His internal training for six months consisted of beating his palm on a large basin full of water.
After six months, the boy was granted a visit to his parents.
During dinner that night, with candles bringing light to the house, an argument was heard between the father and the child, who slapped a wooden kitchen table, breaking the legs and the middle.
This teaches us the results of cultivating with discipline this powerful Iron Palm chi (Qi) storage training method.

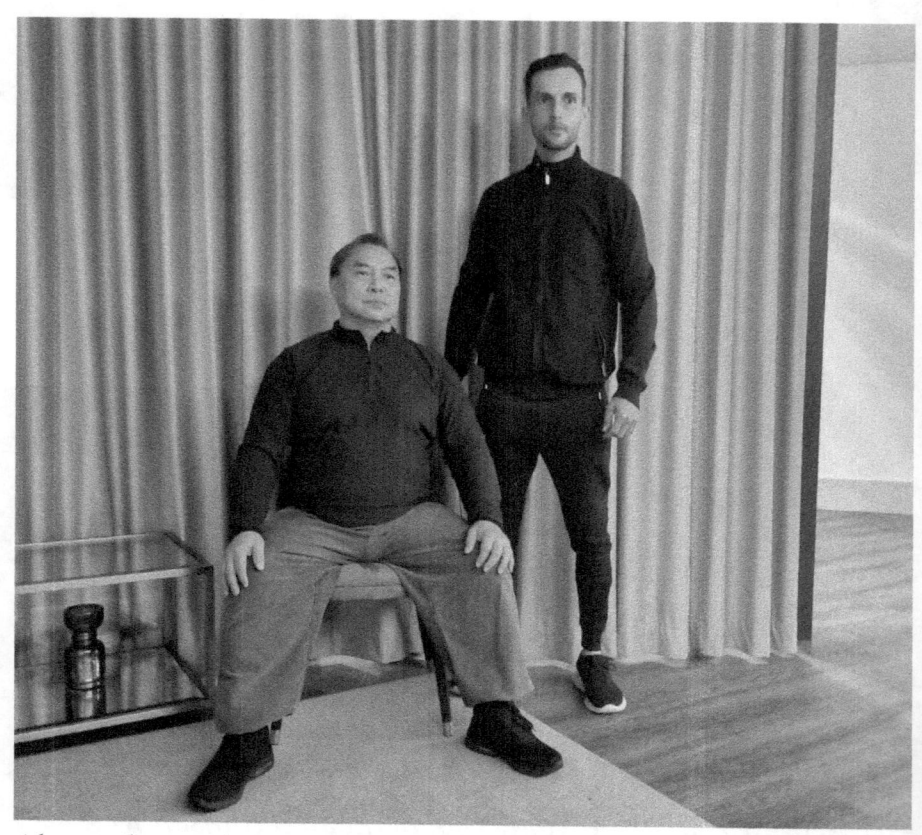

About the author

After 22 years of studies, Sifu Zeca da Vila Barbosa, a historian and master in Wing Chun, Hung Gar, Tai Chi Chuan, Acupuncture and Chi Kung (Qi Gong), explains part of the secret kept in his clan and invites sincere lovers to immerse themselves in the noble art, test themselves and seek a different way of life.

Sifu Zeca is a direct disciple of Grandmaster Lai from Hong Kong and belongs to one of the most traditional families within Kung Fu and his knowledge and traditional method attracts the attention of practitioners from all over the world. Currently, Sifu Zeca lives in Portugal, maintaining the tradition of accepting only a few disciples, immersing them in a very deep layer within kung fu with its traditions such as the Chinese name that the student receives and the stone seal after doing the Bai Sii (tea ceremony between disciple and master). After that comes the Jiu Phai (the traditional Chinese plaque given to the student as authorization to teach) in addition to cultures such as Chinese medicine, painting, Bonsai Dim Mak (touch of death), Iron Shirt and Iron Palm. Sifu Zeca does not teach in academies, only sincere students (disciples) who are accepted or not after a conversation and a cup of tea, and seek commitment to the art. He has been promoting seminars all over the world. His disciples who teach openly are synonymous with great teachers of REAL TRADITIONAL KUNG FU.

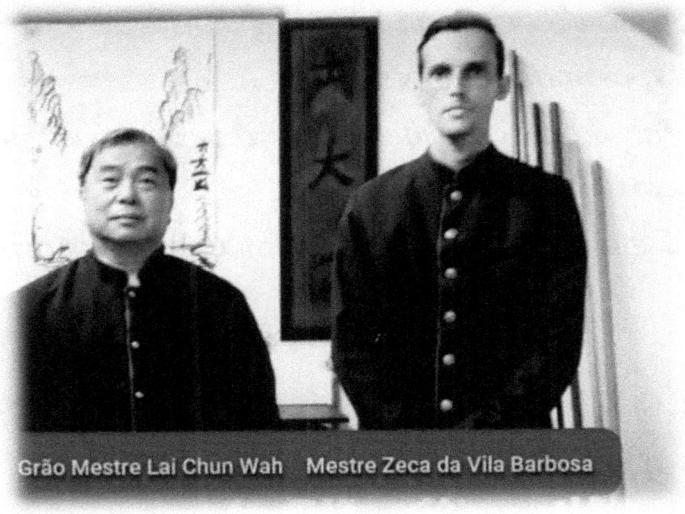

Grão Mestre Lai Chun Wah   Mestre Zeca da Vila Barbosa

Chapter structure:

1. Introduction: What is Iron Palm?
2. Origin and History of the Iron Palm Technique in Kung Fu
3. The Fundamentals of Iron Palm
4. Philosophical and Spiritual Aspects of Iron Palm
5. Physical Preparation for Iron Palm Training
6. Warm-up and Care to Avoid Injuries
7. Traditional Equipment Used in Training
8. Basic Training: First Steps in Iron Palm
9. Advanced Training: Strengthening the Body and Mind
10. Internal Aspects: Energy Development (Qi) in Iron Palm
11. The Connection between Breathing and Strength
12. Nutrition and Diet for Iron Palm Practitioners
13. Success Stories and Inspiring Stories
14. Types and Trainings of Iron Palm
15. The Ethics of Using Iron Palm: Responsibility and Respect
16. Conclusion: How Iron Palm Can Transform Your Life

Chapter 1: Introduction – What is Iron Palm?

Iron Palm is one of the most iconic and respected techniques in traditional Kung Fu, known for its effectiveness and combination of physical strength and internal energy (Qi). It is an intensive training method that transforms the practitioner's hands into powerful tools, capable of withstanding impacts and generating destructive force without compromising health or physical integrity.

This practice dates back centuries of development within Chinese martial arts, and is often associated with styles such as Shaolin and Wudang. Iron Palm is not just a physical technique; it is a path to self-knowledge, emotional balance and spiritual strengthening.

Training requires dedication, patience and a methodical approach. It involves not only physical exercises such as strengthening tendons and bones, but also internal practices that stimulate the flow of Qi throughout the body. Mastery of Iron Palm is achieved when the practitioner is able to combine technique, mental concentration and bodily harmony.

In this guide, we will explore all aspects of this fascinating art: from its history and philosophy to practical training methods. You will learn the importance of breathing, nutrition, and traditional tools used to strengthen your hands. More than that, you will discover how this technique can transform not only your body, but also your mind.

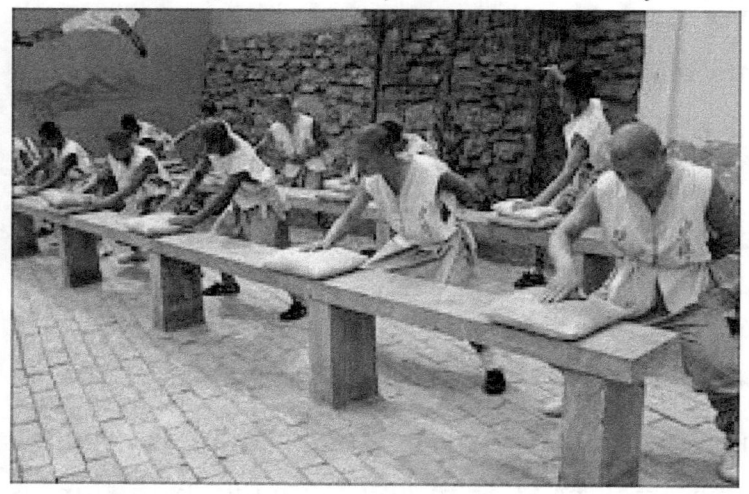

Chapter 2: Origin and History of the Iron Palm Technique in Kung Fu

The Iron Palm technique has deep roots in Chinese martial arts traditions, particularly within the Shaolin and Wudang monasteries. The practice dates back over a thousand years, when Shaolin monks began developing methods to strengthen the body and spirit, seeking protection in times of conflict and spiritual expansion.

According to legend, the monks used the Iron Palm for both self-defense and spiritual pursuits, believing that mastery of the technique increased the flow of life energy, or Qi, throughout the body. During the Tang Dynasty (618-907), Kung Fu flourished as a highly respected art, and the Iron Palm became one of the most impressive aspects of martial training.

Ancient practitioners trained using bags of rice, sand, and metal, applying gradually increasing pressure to harden their hands and prepare the body to absorb impacts. Furthermore, many historical records suggest that the training was not just physical: it included meditative and breathing practices to channel internal energy. Over time, the technique was passed down from generation to generation, evolving to meet the needs of warriors and martial artists. Iron Palm also inspired the development of other combat styles and remains relevant today, both as a method of self-defense and as a discipline for mental and physical strengthening. The combination of tradition, efficiency, and spiritual connection makes Iron Palm one of the most fascinating and enduring techniques in Kung Fu. In the next chapter, we will explore the fundamentals of this extraordinary practice, with a focus on its importance and impact in the modern day.

Chapter 3: The Fundamentals of Iron Palm

The foundation of the Iron Palm technique is the integration of physical strength, internal energy (Qi) and mental discipline. These fundamentals are essential for any practitioner who wishes to master this ancient art.

Physical Strengthening

Iron Palm training requires the gradual development of resistance in the hands, wrists and forearms. Practice begins with the use of materials such as bags of rice or sand, which are progressively replaced by iron grains or harder surfaces. This strengthens not only the muscles, but also the tendons and bones, preparing the hands to withstand impacts without injury.

Breathing and Internal Energy

Breathing is the heart of internal training. Techniques such as Qigong (chi kung see our guides) help practitioners channel and accumulate energy in the dantian (the energy center located below the navel). This energy is then directed to the hands during strikes, amplifying the impact and protecting the body from damage.

Conditioning Practices

- **Massage and Soaking:** Hands are often soaked in medicinal herbs or massaged with specific oils to improve blood circulation and speed recovery.

- **Repetitive Strikes:** Repetition is essential to develop strength and precision. Each strike must be accompanied by mental focus and postural alignment.

Mental Focus and Concentration

More than a physical technique, Iron Palm is a mental practice. Concentration is essential to synchronize the mind with the body, ensuring that each movement is efficient and powerful. Meditation, often combined with training, helps the practitioner achieve deep states of focus and inner calm.

Mastering the fundamentals is the first step to progressing in Iron Palm. In the next chapter, we will discuss how philosophical and spiritual aspects complement this technical learning.

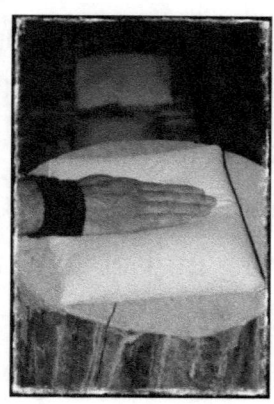

Chapter 4: Philosophical and Spiritual Aspects of Iron Palm

Iron Palm is much more than a combat technique; it incorporates philosophical and spiritual aspects deeply rooted in the tradition of Chinese martial arts. Its purpose is not only to strengthen the body, but also to harmonize the mind and spirit, promoting inner balance and self-discovery.

The Philosophy of Discipline

Iron Palm training requires patience and dedication. Progress is gradual, teaching practitioners the importance of persistence and acceptance of their own limitations. This process reflects the Taoist philosophy of fluidity and adaptation, where strength arises not from rigidity, but from resilience.

Connection with Qi

The spiritual aspects of the technique are closely linked to the manipulation of vital energy, Qi. Through practices such as meditation and controlled breathing, practitioners learn to accumulate and direct this energy, achieving a state of internal harmony. This balance is essential for strikes to have maximum force without causing damage to the body.

Harmony and Responsibility

A core principle of Chinese martial arts is the ethical use of force. Iron Palm is not taught for the purpose of aggression, but as a form of self-defense and personal growth. Masters emphasize that true strength lies in the ability to avoid conflict and use the technique responsibly.

Personal Development

The practice of Iron Palm has transformative effects:

• Strengthening the mind: Improves focus, reduces stress, and increases emotional resilience.

• Spiritual growth: Promotes self-knowledge and connection with the universe around us.

In the next chapter, we will explore how to prepare the body for Iron Palm training, addressing physical strengthening exercises and preventive care.

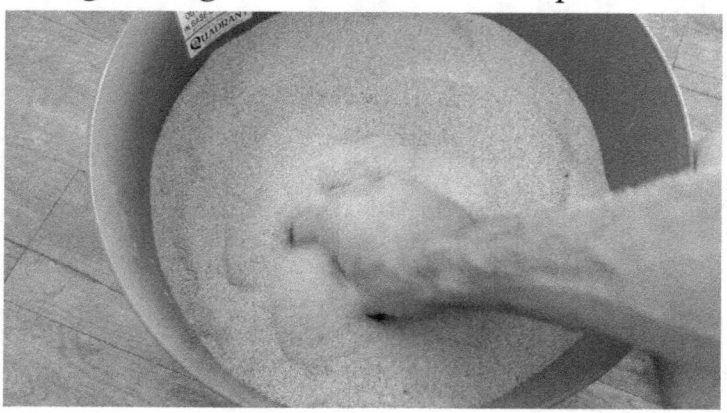

Chapter 5: Physical Preparation for Iron Palm Training

Iron Palm training requires careful physical preparation to ensure that the body is strong and resilient enough to withstand the progressive impact of the practices. This preparation is essential to avoid injury and to ensure the gradual and effective development of the hands, wrists and arms.

Muscle Conditioning

Strengthening the muscles of the hands, forearms and shoulders is an essential step in training. Exercises such as close-fist push-ups, lifting light weights and squeezing rubber balls help to build muscle strength and improve endurance.

Joint Strengthening

The joints of the fingers and wrists bear much of the impact during the exercises. Specific practices, such as using bags of rice and gradually sand or metal, help to condition these areas. Wrist rotation exercises and hand stretches are also essential.

Stretching Routine

Before any practice, a good warm-up is crucial. Stretching movements of the fingers, hands and arms help to increase flexibility and reduce the risk of injury. Stretching the muscles in your torso and legs is also helpful, as many techniques rely on a stable body base.

Core Training

Although the Iron Palm technique focuses on the hands, a strong body base is essential. Exercises such as planks, squats, and twists help build stability and balance. A strong core allows you to transfer the force of your entire body to your hands during strikes.

Protection and Recovery

Iron Palm training should be done progressively. Applying traditional Chinese herbs and oils to your hands helps minimize damage and speeds recovery. In addition, taking regular breaks is essential to allow your body to recover and adapt to the training.

Preparing your body is just the beginning of the journey. In the next chapter, we will discuss how to prevent injuries through proper warm-up and safe Iron Palm training practices.

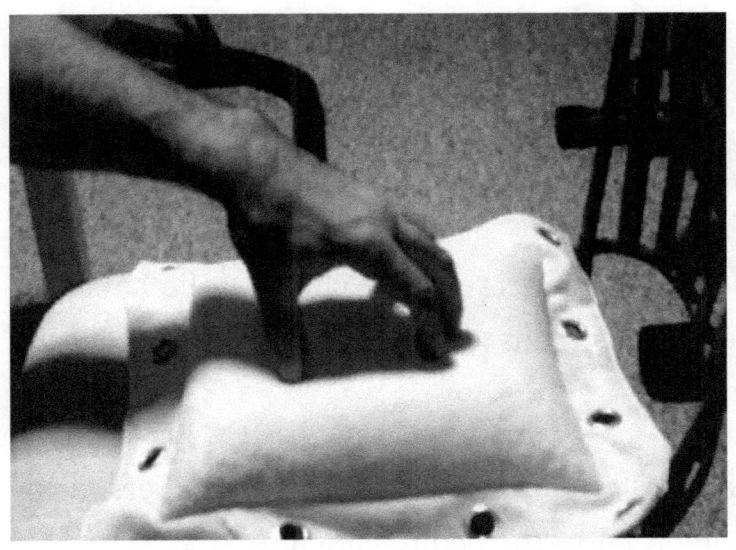

Chapter 6: Warm-up and Injury Prevention

Iron Palm training can be intense, and safety should always be a priority. Proper warm-up and preventive care are essential to minimize the risk of injury and ensure that the body is prepared to withstand the increasing impacts during practice.

The Importance of Warming Up

Warming up prepares the muscles, tendons and joints for training. It improves blood circulation, increases flexibility and reduces stiffness, making the body more resistant to injuries.

Essential Warm-Up Exercises:

1. Circular movements with the wrists and fingers: Promotes flexibility in the joints.

2. Moderate push-ups with the palms of the hands on the floor: Strengthens the wrists and warms up the arm muscles.

3. Dynamic stretches: Stretching the shoulders, arms and spine prepares the body as a whole.

4. Hand massage: Applying light pressure to the fingers and palms activates circulation and relaxes the tissues.

Safe Training Techniques

• Progression: Never move directly onto materials such as iron or wood without starting with softer surfaces, such as rice bags.

• Moderate repetitions: Do not overdo the number of blows per session; increase gradually as your body adapts.

• Correct posture: Maintain body alignment, with feet firmly planted, to distribute the impact safely.

• Remember to cultivate patience and peace of mind.

Post-Workout Care

After each session, relaxation and recovery practices help the body heal and strengthen itself.

- Soaking in medicinal herbs: Helps relieve inflammation and accelerate tissue regeneration. (Jow Note: Many families or clans have their own hand-to-hand technique, like us at Ning Nam Tong)

- Gentle stretching: Reduces accumulated muscle tension.

- Therapeutic massage: Use traditional balms or oils to promote circulation and reduce pain. Warning Signs

If you experience severe pain, swelling, or persistent numbness in your hands, it is crucial to stop training and seek guidance from a master or health professional.

With safe practices, Iron Palm training becomes an enriching and injury-free journey. In the next chapter, we will explore the traditional equipment used to develop strength and endurance in this technique.

Chapter 7: Traditional Equipment Used in Training

Iron Palm training is deeply rooted in traditional methods that involve the use of simple but effective equipment. These devices have been developed over centuries and are designed to condition the hands in a progressive and safe manner.

Training Bags

Training bags are one of the most iconic tools in Iron Palm. They evolve in terms of density and content as the practitioner progresses through the training.

• Rice Bags: Used in the early stages to strengthen the sensitivity and muscles of the hands.

• Sand Bags: Introduced in the intermediate stage to increase endurance and strength.

• Iron Bags: Intended for advanced practitioners, they toughen the hands and tendons.

Wooden Poles and Posts

Wooden posts, often covered with leather or fabric, are used to train accuracy and impact. The practice involves repetitive strikes to condition the palms and increase tolerance to shock. Stone Plates and Bricks

These objects help develop finger strength and precision of movement. Exercises usually involve pressing or breaking the plates, always with proper control and technique.

Wooden or Metal Rollers

Used to massage and strengthen the fingers and palms, these rollers help improve circulation and endurance. They are often combined with medicinal oils or balms.

Herbs and Recovery Tools

In addition to training equipment, traditional tools for soaking the hands in medicinal liquids are essential.

- Bowls of Medicinal Herbs: Used to relieve pain and promote recovery.

- Balms and Oils: Applied after training to protect the skin and reduce inflammation.

Simplicity of Equipment

The use of simple equipment reflects the essence of Kung Fu: the skill of the practitioner always surpasses the sophistication of the tools. The focus is on gradual development, patience and respect for one's own body. With an understanding of the traditional apparatus, we are ready to explore the basic Iron Palm training in the next chapter, which forms the basis for future advancements.

Chapter 8: Basic Training - Getting Started in Iron Palm

Basic Iron Palm training is the foundation for progressing in this powerful technique. It involves simple, controlled exercises that strengthen the hands, improve coordination, and introduce the fundamental principles of the practice.

Basic Training Principles

1. Progressivity: Start with soft materials, such as bags of rice or sand, and gradually increase intensity.

2. Focus on Breathing: Each strike should be accompanied by deep, controlled breaths to maximize strength and protect the body.

3. Consistency: Progress comes with regular practice, not with overexertion in a single day.

Essential Beginning Exercises

1. Palm Strikes

• Purpose: Strengthen the surface of the hand.

- How to Do It: Lightly strike a bag of rice with an open palm. Start with 10 to 20 repetitions per hand and gradually increase.

- Tip: Keep your fingers aligned and use your breath to channel the energy.

2. Finger Pressing Movements

- Purpose: Strengthen your fingers for precise punching.

- How to Do It: Press down on a flat, firm surface (such as a table or wooden board) with your fingers extended.

- Tip: Avoid tensing your wrists; focus only on your fingers.

3. Massage Conditioning

- Purpose: Prepare your muscles and improve circulation.

- How to Do It: After each training session, massage your hands using medicated oils to relieve tension.

Posture and Alignment

Proper posture is vital to ensure the safety and effectiveness of your training.

- Keep your feet firmly planted on the floor, shoulder-width apart.

- Relax your shoulders and keep your spine straight.

- Focus on balancing your body as you apply force to your palms.

Closing Ritual

The closing of each session is as important as the training itself. Practice slow, deep breathing for a few minutes to relax your body and restore your Qi. With a solid foundation in the basic exercises, the practitioner will be ready to advance to more challenging levels. In the next chapter, we will cover advanced training and how it expands on the skills learned in the initial stages.

Chapter 9: Advanced Training – Strengthening the Body and Mind

Once the fundamentals have been mastered, the Iron Palm practitioner can advance to more challenging techniques that not only strengthen the hands but also develop mental toughness and energy control. These advanced trainings require constant dedication and discipline.

Evolution in the Use of Equipment

1. Iron Bag Strikes

- Objective: To toughen the hands and fingers.

- How to do it: Strike a bag filled with iron grains or small pieces of metal. Start with short sessions and gradually increase the duration.

- Tip: Always apply protective oils before and after training.

2. Breaking Materials

- Objective: To demonstrate strength and precision.

- How to do it: Practice breaking materials such as blocks of wood or bricks with precise strikes.

- Tip: Concentrate on technique and mental focus before executing the strike.

3. Stone Slab Training

- Objective: To strengthen fingers and wrists. • How to do it: Press the plates with your fingers, applying gradual force. This exercise strengthens the tendons and improves control.

Deepening Qi and Breathing

Control of internal energy (Qi) is vital in advanced training.

- Directed Breathing: Coordinate your inhalation and exhalation with your strikes to maximize energy transfer.

- Active Meditation: During training, visualize the flow of Qi going from the dantian to your hands, strengthening the impact.

Mental Resilience

At the advanced level, the practitioner must cultivate a resilient mindset, capable of withstanding physical discomfort without losing concentration. Regular meditation practice helps develop focus and emotional control.

Intensified Recovery Routine

As the intensity of training increases, recovery becomes even more essential.

- Herbal Soaks: Herbs such as ginseng and Chinese angelica help revitalize the tissues.

- Specific Stretches: Spend more time stretching your hands and wrists to avoid muscle stiffness.

With advanced training, the practitioner can achieve an impressive level of strength and control. In the next chapter, we will delve into the internal aspects of the technique, exploring how internal energy and Qi play a crucial role in Iron Palm.

Chapter 10: Internal Aspects – Energy (Qi) Development in Iron Palm

One of the deepest secrets of the Iron Palm technique lies in the internal aspects, especially in the mastery of Qi, or vital energy. Internal training is what differentiates a simple physical strike from a powerful technique that harmonizes body, mind and spirit.

The Role of Qi in Iron Palm

Qi is the vital force that flows throughout the body. In Iron Palm practice, it is directed to the hands, strengthening the strikes and protecting the practitioner from internal injuries.

- Increases the effectiveness of strikes: Qi amplifies physical strength.

- Promotes internal resilience: Protects organs and tissues from repetitive impacts.

Practices for Developing Qi

1. Specific Qigong for Iron Palm (see our material on chi kung or qi gong)

- Objective: Channel and accumulate energy in the dantian (energy center in the abdomen).

- How to do it:

1. Adopt a firm position, such as the horse stance.

2. Inhale deeply through your nose, visualizing the energy flowing down to your dantian.

3. Exhale slowly through your mouth, directing the Qi to your palms.

4. Repeat for 10 to 20 minutes daily.

2. Guided Meditation

- Purpose: Strengthen focus and the mind-body connection.

- How to do it:

1. Sit in a quiet place and close your eyes.

2. Focus on your breathing and visualize the Qi flowing through the meridians to your hands.

3. Practice visualization for 15 minutes before beginning physical training.

3. Dynamic Breathing Techniques

- Purpose: Increase the flow of energy during punches.

- How to do it:

1. Inhale deeply before the punch.

2. Exhale forcefully as you strike, releasing the Qi through your hands.

Internal Balance and Health

Internal training is not just about strength. It also promotes overall health and emotional balance. Practitioners report:

- Reduced stress and increased mental calm.

- Improved circulation and overall vitality.

- Strengthened immunity through the harmonious flow of Qi.

Qi Care

Overexertion can deplete Qi. Therefore, it is crucial to balance internal training with adequate rest and restorative practices, such as massage and the use of tonifying herbs.

By mastering the internal aspects, the practitioner is prepared to integrate mind and body in a unique way, elevating their technique to an exceptional level. In the next chapter, we will explore the connection between breath and strength, delving deeper into the importance of this fundamental element in Iron Palm.

Chapter 11. The Connection Between Breathing and Strength

In the practice of Iron Palm, breathing is the bridge that connects the physical body to internal energy (Qi). The way the practitioner breathes during the exercises directly influences the strength, precision and resistance of the strikes.

The Importance of Breathing in Kung Fu

Controlled breathing is not just a technical element; it is the foundation for channeling energy and maintaining internal balance. Each inhalation and exhalation synchronized with the movements allows:

• Maximizing force: Breathing propels the strike, releasing accumulated energy.

• Minimizing physical wear and tear: Controls the flow of oxygen and maintains resistance.

• Protecting the body: Reduces negative impact on muscles and joints.

Essential Breathing Techniques

1. Deep Abdominal Breathing

• Objective: Accumulate Qi in the dantian and stabilize energy.

• How to do it:

1. Inhale deeply through the nose, expanding the abdomen.

2. Hold your breath for 2 to 3 seconds, concentrating your Qi.

3. Exhale slowly through your mouth, feeling the energy flow through your hands.

2. Explosive Breathing

• Objective: Release maximum force during a strike.

• How to do it:

1. Inhale quickly before striking.

2. Exhale forcefully, producing a controlled sound ("ha" or "sss"), releasing Qi at the moment of impact.

3. Cyclic Breathing

• Objective: Sustain continuous strikes without losing energy.

• How to do it:

1. Inhale rhythmically between strikes.

2. Exhale briefly and precisely with each strike.

Integrating Breathing with Movements

One of the most valuable skills of Iron Palm is synchronizing breathing and movement. The practitioner learns to:

• Inhale while preparing for a strike.

• Exhale at the moment of impact.

- Maintain controlled breathing in prolonged sessions, balancing strength and focus.

Physical and Mental Benefits

- Physical: Improved lung capacity, core strength, and increased endurance.

- Mental: Controlled breathing reduces stress and increases mental clarity, promoting a state of calm even under pressure.

Practical Training

Spend 5 to 10 minutes at the beginning of each session practicing breathing exercises, gradually integrating them into your strikes and movements. This practice creates a solid foundation for complete mastery of the technique.

In the next chapter, we will explore how nutrition and diet play a crucial role in the performance and recovery of Iron Palm practitioners.

Chapter 12: Nutrition and Diet for Iron Palm Practitioners

Nutrition plays a vital role in Iron Palm training, directly influencing strength, endurance, and recovery. A balanced diet strengthens the body, supports overall health, and promotes the circulation of Qi.

Basic Nutrition Principles for Practitioners

1. Sustained Energy: Whole foods provide long-lasting energy for intense training.

2. Internal Balance: The diet should promote harmony in the body, avoiding foods that cause inflammation or block the flow of energy.

3. Accelerated Recovery: Certain foods and herbs help repair tissue and strengthen bones.

Essential Foods for Training

1. Protein

• Necessary for muscle building and recovery.

• Sources: Eggs, fish, tofu, chicken, lentils.

2. Whole Grains

• Provide sustained energy during training.

- Sources: Brown rice, quinoa, oats, whole-wheat bread.

3. Vegetables

- Rich in vitamins, minerals, and antioxidants to protect cells.

- Sources: Spinach, broccoli, carrots, kale.

4. Healthy Fats

- Help with energy production and brain function.

- Sources: Avocado, nuts, olive oil, chia seeds.

5. Fruits

- Provides quick energy and promotes hydration.

- Sources: Bananas, apples, oranges, berries.

Chinese Herbs and Supplements

Traditional Chinese medicine suggests herbs that strengthen Qi and speed recovery:

- Ginseng: Increases energy and vitality.

- Angelica sinensis (Dong Quai): Promotes blood circulation and speeds healing.

- Goji Berries: Rich in antioxidants and great for immunity.

- Hydration and Fluids

Staying hydrated is essential for Qi circulation and overall health.

- Drink water regularly throughout the day.

- Green or herbal tea are great for detoxifying the body.

Foods to Avoid

1. Fried and ultra-processed foods: Can cause inflammation.

2. Refined sugars: Drain energy throughout the day.

3. Alcoholic beverages: Unbalance Qi and slow recovery.

Meal Planning

- Pre-workout: Light foods rich in carbohydrates and a little protein.

- Post-workout: Focus on proteins and healthy fats for recovery.

- During the day: Maintain balanced meals and avoid long periods without eating.

A proper diet enhances training results and helps the practitioner reach higher levels in Iron Palm. In the next chapter, we will learn about success stories and inspiring stories of masters of this legendary technique.

Chapter 13: Success Stories and Inspirational Stories

The Iron Palm technique has been practiced for centuries, and many masters have distinguished themselves with their extraordinary feats. These inspiring stories show the power of dedication and consistent training, motivating new practitioners to follow suit.

Legendary Masters

1. Wang Xu, the Stone Breaker

Wang Xu is a legendary figure in Chinese martial arts, known for his ability to shatter massive boulders with a single palm strike. He began his training at the age of 10, dedicating himself to traditional methods and internal strengthening through meditation. His fame led him to be called the "Invincible Hand" in his home village.

2. Master Li Feng and the Defense of the Temple

During the Ming Dynasty, the Shaolin Temple was frequently attacked. Master Li Feng, an advanced practitioner of the Iron Palm, led the defense with his incredible ability to repel invaders using only his hands. His story is told as an example of courage and martial skill.

3. Chen Bao, the Inner Energy Pacifist

Chen Bao dedicated his life to training internally in Iron Palm. Despite possessing impressive strength, he chose to resolve conflicts peacefully. He inspired many by showing that true strength lies in self-control and the responsible use of skills.

Recent Stories

1. Modern Practitioner Who Overcame Limits

A modern example is Li Wei, who excelled in Iron Palm training after an accident that nearly left him disabled. He used the practice as rehabilitation, showing that discipline and determination can overcome even physical adversity.

2. Iron Palm in Modern Sports

Mixed martial arts athletes have adapted Iron Palm techniques to improve strength, precision and endurance, showing how this ancient practice continues to have relevance in the modern world.

Lessons from Masters and Practitioners

• Dedication: The greatest practitioners of Iron Palm dedicated their lives to methodical training.

• Respect for Traditions: Many emphasize the importance of preserving traditional methods and values.

• Resilience: Stories of overcoming adversity show that anyone can progress with persistence and focus.

These inspiring stories demonstrate that Iron Palm is more than a technique; it is a path to self-development. In the next chapter, we will discuss the ethics of using Iron Palm, a crucial topic for any practitioner.

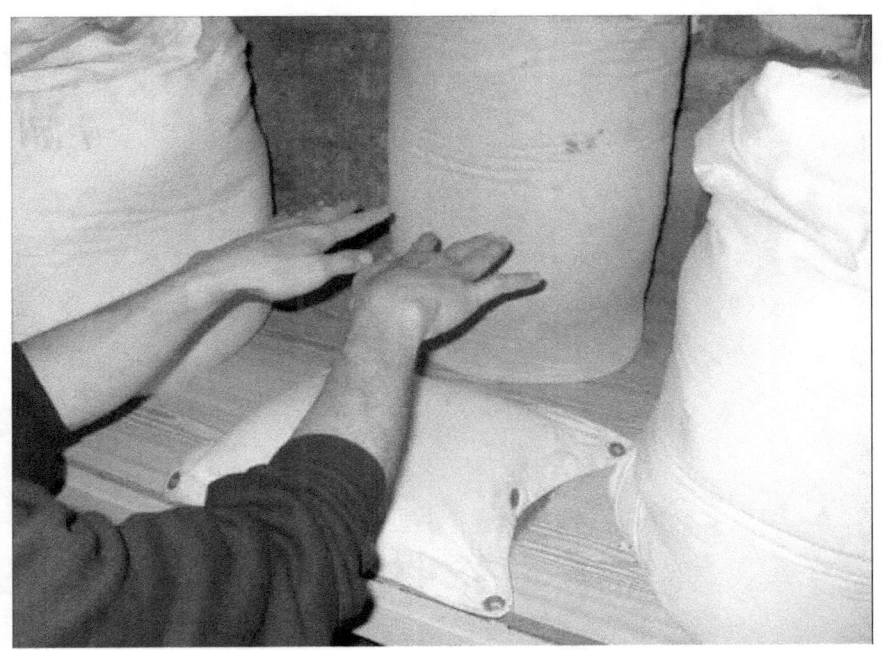

Chapter 14: Iron palm training and techniques.

Note: I preserve the quality of the images taken from the original books

Northern Iron Palm: Composed of three stages: palm, back of the hands and knife of the hand, the most common and published until the research points out.

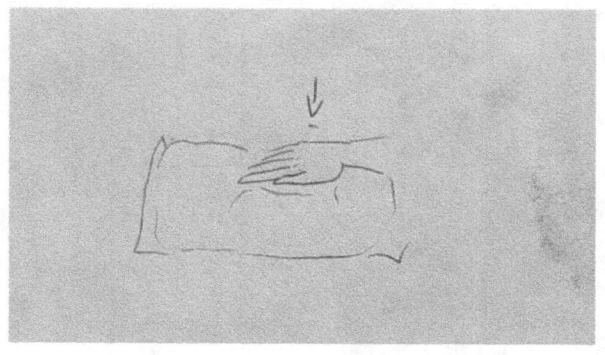

Palm

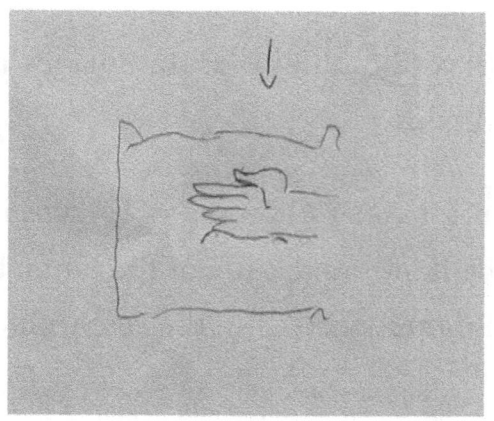

Coast hand

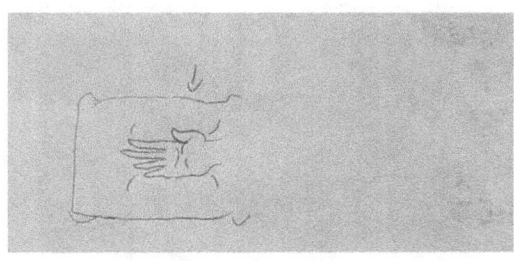

Knife hand

Zhu Li Kan's palm, the demon's palm: This technique consists of initial training of attacks with fingertips in a container with sand and pepper to increase the flow of chi (Qi). It penetrates if the fingers are already trained, fills the hands with sand and pepper. Others use iron balls without pepper and punches the bag in front, then releases the sand or iron that the fingers captured when penetrating. This technique is used in addition to the sand and iron bag of the traditional northern palm. It is very powerful and restricted only to Zhu Li Kan's misunderstandings, but due to the friendship presented here.

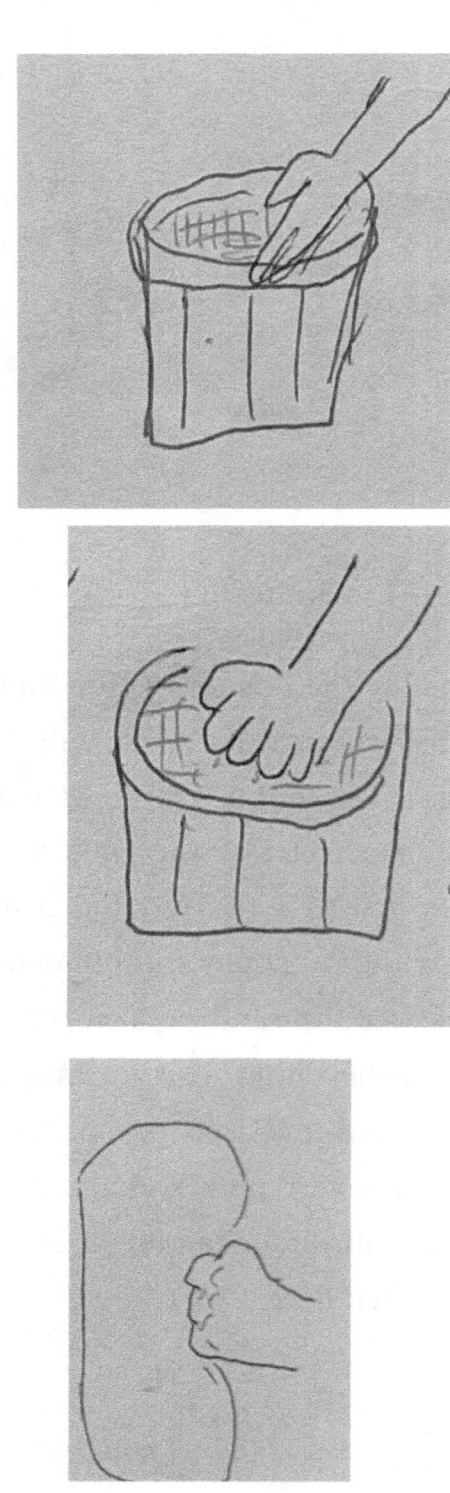

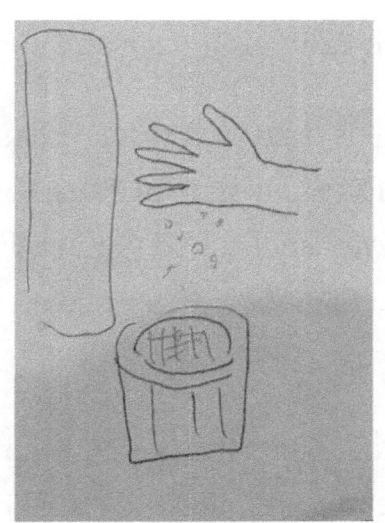

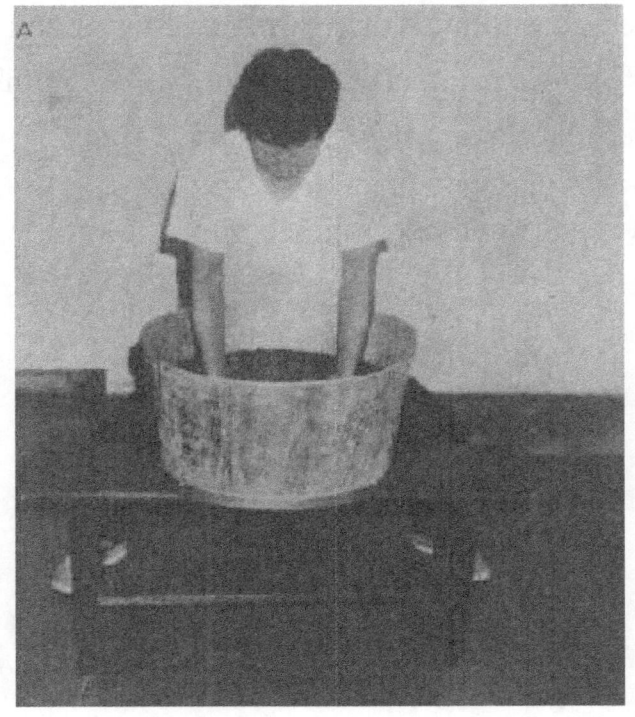

Hung Gar Iron Palm or Tiger Iron Palm

This technique is used by a triad or Hung Men who practice the Hung Gar style of Tang Fong and Chow Wing Tak previously trained with boiling sand and boiling oil like the movie "tiger claws" with Bolo Yueng

This technique follows the three initial northern techniques (see above) plus the crane beak technique, then pushes the sandbag forward using the wrist impact and tiger claw and then uses the tiger claw to capture and pull back using the diaphragm and throat sound "huuuurr" tamp practitioners throw sandbags to each other to capture with the tiger claw.

This iron palm training when completed is very powerful.

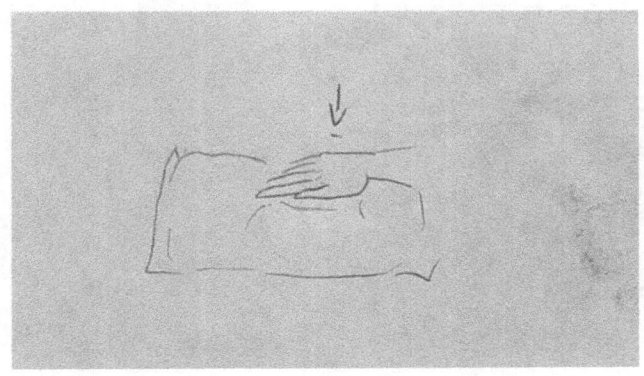

Palm

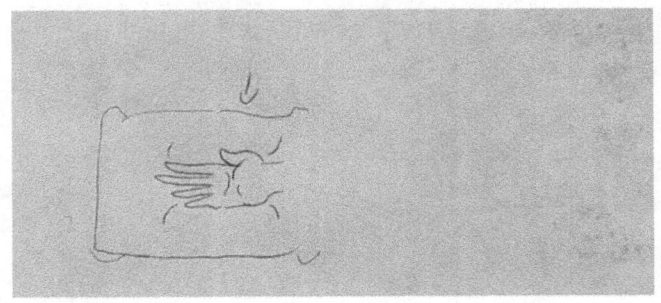

hand coast

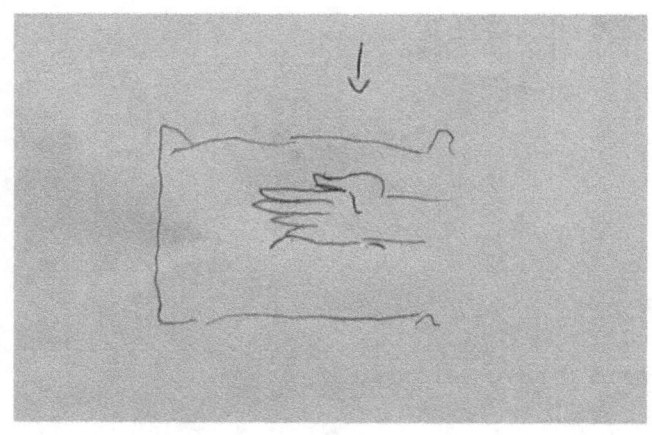

hand knife

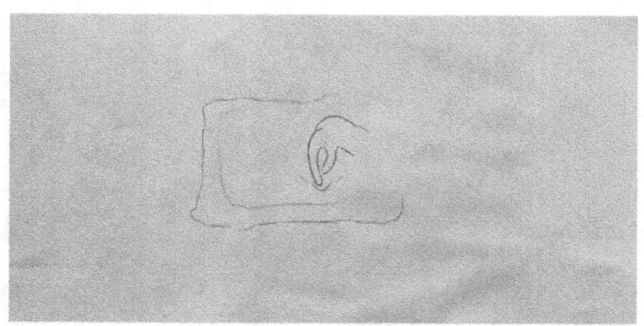

Crane

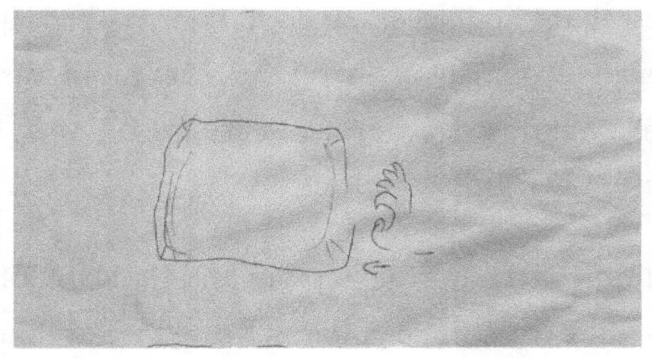

Tiger claw pushing forward

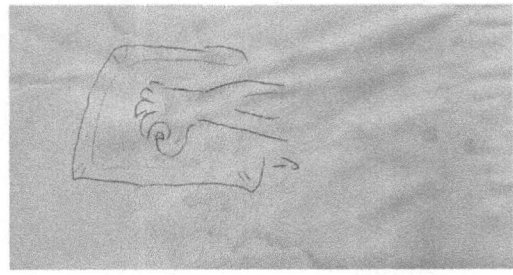

Tiger claw captures and pulls back

Iron palm of the ancient branches of Wing Chun of the Chinese mafia

In this branch after 20 years of studies only 5 students of Ip Man, Bruce Lee's master, taught this technique. The rest that I had access to do not derive from Ip Man, some from Pan Nam, others from more "discreet" lineages that do not accept Westerners, but they are still very powerful.

In addition to the northern palm and the palm of Zhu Li Kan, they train the iron palm using angles that Wing Chun has in its characteristics, dodging the opponent's attack and attacking strategic points such as the eye, throat and diaphragm..

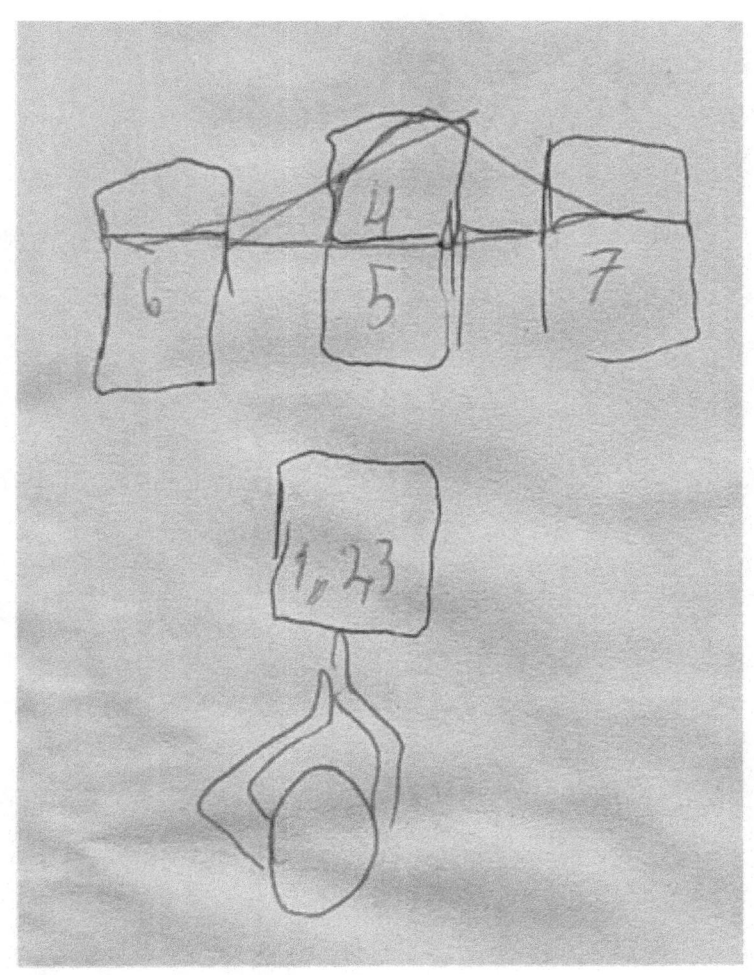

Posture in front of the 4 bags

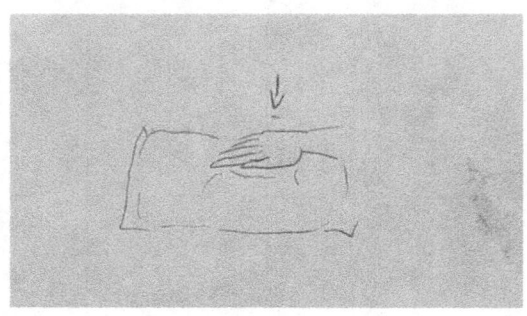

Palm

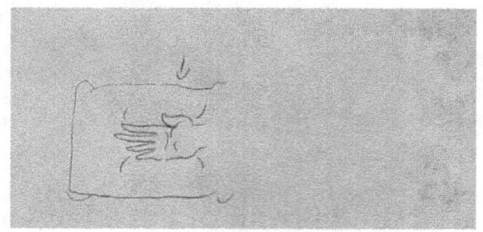

Hand Coast

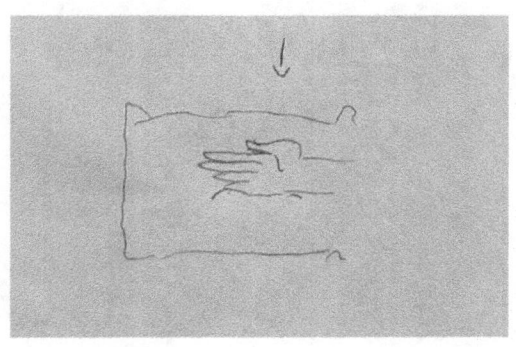

Knife hand

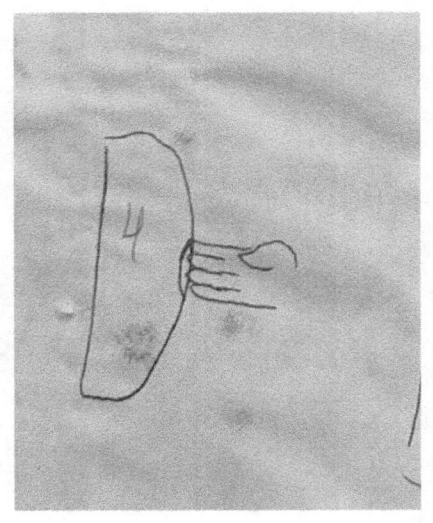

Biu Sau fingertips

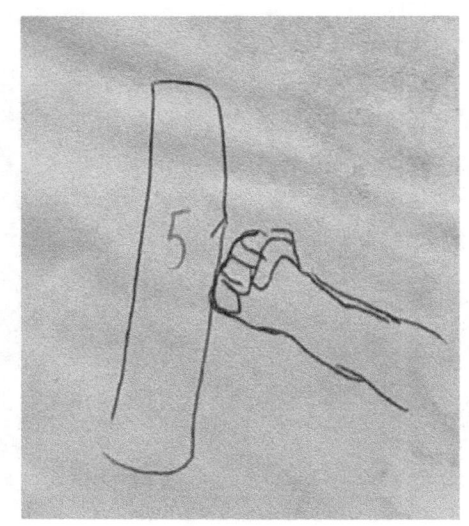

punch

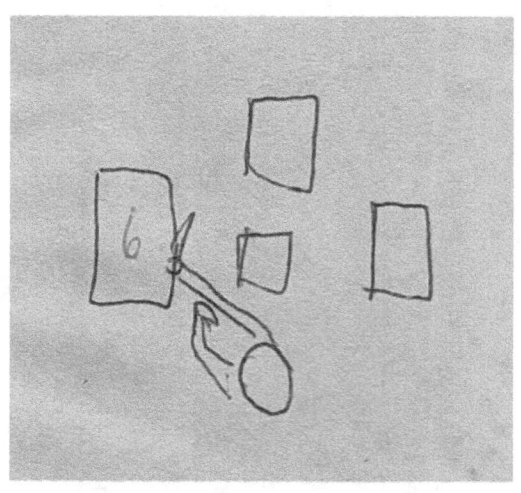

Jalm side palm

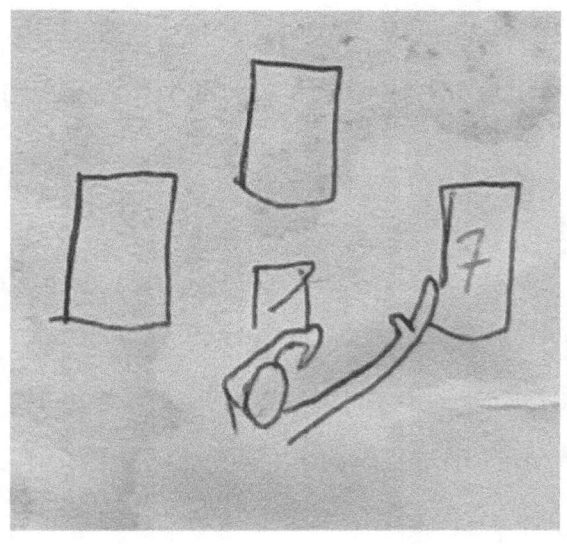

Fak Sau

Chapter 15: The Ethics of Using Iron Palm – Responsibility and Respect

1. Iron Palm is a powerful technique that requires a rigorous ethical approach. Traditional masters emphasize that by acquiring this skill, the practitioner also assumes a great moral responsibility.
2. Fundamental Principles of Ethics
3. 1. Self-control: Mastery of Iron Palm is measured not only by physical strength, but by the ability to control when and how to use it.
4. 2. Defense, not aggression: The technique should only be used as a last resort, never to start a conflict.

5. Respect for your opponent: Even in combat situations, it is important to treat your opponent with dignity.

The Kung Fu Code of Conduct

Masters often teach that strength should be balanced by compassion. The primary goal of training is not to inflict harm, but to protect oneself and others while maintaining peace.

Lessons in Responsibility

- Avoid ostentation: Demonstrating power or using technique to impress others disrespects your principles.

- Teach with care: A master must assess the character of his students before passing on the technique.

- Beware of excess: Intense practice can cause physical and emotional harm if conducted without balance.

Ethical Use Cases

1. Self-defense: Practitioners who have used the technique to protect themselves from physical attacks.

2. Protection of others: Accounts of masters who have intervened in dangerous situations to save others.

3. Transmission of wisdom: Masters who used the practice as a tool for personal transformation for their students, promoting discipline and self-knowledge.

Risks of Improper Use

1. Arrogance: Abusing the technique can lead to unnecessary conflicts.

2. Permanent injuries: Reckless use can cause serious harm to both the practitioner and the opponent.

3. Disruption of internal balance: Improper use can generate emotional and energetic imbalances.

The Path of the True Master

A true practitioner of the Iron Palm understands that the greatest power lies in not having to use it. Self-control, inner peace and the search for harmony are the values that define a master.

Understanding ethics is essential for any practitioner. In the final chapter, we will conclude the guide by exploring how the Iron Palm can transform your life physically, mentally and spiritually.

Chapter 15: Conclusion – How the Iron Palm Can Transform Your Life

The practice of the Iron Palm transcends the limits of a martial technique. It is a journey of self-discovery, discipline and balance that profoundly impacts the practitioner's life, both physically and spiritually.

The Physical and Mental Benefits

- Physical Strength: With consistent training, the hands, wrists, and body as a whole become more resilient.

- Energy Balance: The practice of Qi harmonizes the body, improving overall health and longevity.

- Mental Clarity: The meditation and focus required by the technique strengthen the mind, reducing stress and increasing concentration.

Spiritual Transformation

Iron Palm is not just a physical exercise; it is a spiritual path. By learning to master one's internal energy, the practitioner discovers the balance between strength and serenity, power and compassion.

Daily Applications

The principles of Iron Palm, such as self-control, patience, and persistence, apply to all aspects of life. Whether at work, in relationships, or in personal challenges, these lessons offer valuable tools for facing adversity with calm and resilience.

A Legacy to Be Preserved

As we conclude this guide, it is important to remember that Iron Palm is more than a technique; it is a cultural legacy that carries centuries of wisdom. By practicing it ethically and respectfully, you become part of this tradition, contributing to its preservation and growth. This guide is just the beginning of your journey. Practice regularly, seek out experienced masters and deepen your knowledge of both the physical and internal aspects of the technique. Iron Palm is an art that rewards those who dedicate themselves body and soul, transforming their lives for the better.

We at Ning Nam Tong can help you with this through Sifu Zeca from Vila Barbosa (Lai Hop Long) to purchase materials, bags and Jow, the traditional herbal oil. Email: zecakf@hotmail.com WhatApp +351966794913

The strength is in your hands — and the journey continues.

Sifu Zeca da Vila Barbosa (Lai Hop Long)

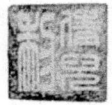